Intermittent Fasting Recipes

The Perfect Guide to Begin Intermittent Fasting in a Balanced and Effective Way and Practical guide for weight loss to lose 10 pounds

(Health Benefits Intermittent Fasting for Weight Loss)

Eduardo Pittman

Published by Jason Thawne Publishing House

© Eduardo Pittman

Intermittent Fasting Recipes: The Perfect Guide to Begin Intermittent Fasting in a Balanced and Effective Way and Practical guide for weight loss to lose 10 pounds

(Health Benefits Intermittent Fasting for Weight Loss)

All Rights Reserved

ISBN 978-1-989749-64-7

This document is geared towards providing exact and reliable information in regards to the topic and issue covered. The publication is sold with the idea that the publisher isn't required to render accounting, officially permitted, or otherwise, qualified services. If advice is necessary, legal or even professional, a practiced individual in the profession should be ordered.

- From a Declaration of Principles which was accepted and approved equally by a Committee of the American Bar Association and a Committee of Publishers and Associations.

In no way is it legal to reproduce, duplicate, or even transmit any part of this document in either electronic means or in printed format. Recording of this publication is strictly prohibited and any storage of this document isn't allowed unless with proper written permission from the publisher. All rights reserved.

The information provided herein is stated to be truthful and consistent, in that any liability, in terms of inattention or otherwise, by any usage or abuse of any policies, processes, or directions contained within is the solitary and also utter responsibility of the recipient reader. Under no circumstances will any legal responsibility or blame be held against the publisher for any reparation, damages, or monetary loss due to the information herein, either directly or indirectly.

Respective authors own all copyrights not held by the publisher.

The information herein is offered for just informational purposes solely, and is universal as so. The presentation of the information is without contract or any type of guarantee assurance.

The trademarks that are used are without any consent, and also the publication of the trademark is without permission or backing by the trademark owner. All trademarks and brands within this book are for clarifying purposes only and are the owned by the owners themselves, not affiliated with this document.

TABLE OF CONTENTS

Part 1 1

Introduction: 1

What is Intermittent Fasting? 1

The 16/8 Protocol. 3

Healthy chicken pie 3

Ribbon prawns and spaghetti 5

Grilled cauliflower with couscous 6

Chicken wraps 8

Grilled Vegetable Panini with feta 9

Intermediate Level Intermittent Fasting 11

Chili Bean and Bulgur Burger 12

Cauliflower crust pizza 13

Intermittent Fasting Hard Core, Alternative Days 16

Bacon and egg fat bombs (make six servings) 23

Sugar free peanut butter fudge 24

Conclusion 26

Part 2 27

Introduction	28
Overview of The 5:2 Fast Diet	31
5:2 Diet Power Foods	40
Recipes: Under 50 Calories Per Serving	47
Mixed Fruit Salad	48
Baked Pear	50
Broiled Tomato	51
Berry Parfait	54
Smoked Salmon and Tomatoes	55
Veggie Frittata	57
Recipes: 50-100 Calories Per Serving	59
Whole Wheat Blueberry Muffins	59
Baking spray	60
Veggie-Sausage Spinach Cups	62
Low-Calorie Strawberry Granola	64
Chicken-Apple Sausage Patties	68
Multi-Grain English Muffins	70
Orange Juice Cranberry Muffins	74
Potato-Ham Frittata	77

Spray oil 78

Smoked Salmon Breakfast Sandwich 80

Breakfast Bread Pudding 83

Baking spray 84

Apple Crisp 86

Huevos Rancheros 89

Fish Fingers 92

Cooking spray 93

Classic American Breakfast: Bacon, Eggs, and Hash Browns 94

Mini Hash Brown Casseroles 97

Cooking spray 98

Eggs Benedict 100

Overnight Oatmeal 104

Spicy Rice and Egg Bowl 106

Whole Wheat Banana Pancakes 108

Blueberry Oatmeal Pancakes 110

French Toast Waffles 113

Cooking spray 113

Baked Apple Fritter 115

Omelet Wrap 118

Zucchini Breakfast Bread 120

Potato-Sausage Casserole 122

Conclusion 126

About The Author 126

Part 1

Introduction:
What is Intermittent Fasting?

First, let's get one thing clear. Intermittent fasting is not a diet, it is a dieting pattern. Put simply, it is the conscious decision to skip meals on purpose.

The pattern of fasting and feasting generally means that you consume all of your food during a specific period of time rather than a larger window of the day. There are many different ways to introduce intermittent fasting into your lifestyle and you can choose the one that suits you best.

Make sure you consult a doctor or health specialist before you start any program to make sure it is right for you. Women especially should be aware that their female hormone balance might be affected by fasting protocols. Additionally, if you have stomach issues or adrenal fatigue you will need to proceed with caution.

There are different levels of fasting that can be broken down into beginner, intermediate and advanced levels. We will examine plans from all three levels and include recipes for these plans. These can give you an idea of the types of food you will be eating and introduce you to the concept of IF.

Benefits of IF
- Improved mental clarity
- Weight loss
- Increased energy and growth hormone
- Reversal of type 2 diabetes
- Lowered blood cholesterol
- Reduction of inflammation
- Potential prevention of Alzheimer's
- Longer life expectancy
- Activation of cellular cleansing

The 16/8 Protocol.

The logistics behind this IF program is simple. You fast for 16 hours and eat within an 8-hour window. Most people find it easier to fast overnight, skip breakfast and eat their main meal around lunchtime. Fasting between 8 p.m. and 12 midday the following day should work with most schedules.

Here are some healthy recipes that will provide you a great lunch to start your day.

Healthy chicken pie

- 1 cup of mushrooms roughly chopped
- 4 chicken thighs cut into smaller pieces
- 2 tbsp of organic butter
- 2 leeks washed and sliced into pieces
- 1 cup vegetable stock
- Olive oil
- Bunch of spinach leaves
- 4 sheets of filo pastry
- 1 Tsp corn flour
- ½ cup of double cream

Method

1) Preheat oven to 180 degrees centigrade or equivalent
2) Over a high heat melt the butter and add the leeks and mushrooms. When they begin to soften add the chicken thighs and flash fry for a couple of minutes. Add the stock and allow it to simmer gently.
3) Mix corn flour with water until smooth and then add to the pan. Also, add the cream. Bring back to the boil and stir until the sauce thickens. Now add the spinach and wilt the leaves for 30 seconds.
4) Remove the mixture from the stove and place the mixture into a pie dish. Allow to cool for 10 mins.
5) Take the filo pastry in your hands and rough it up a bit. Creased and crumpled lay the pastry on top of the pie filling and repeat with the further sheets.
6) Drizzle the olive oil on the pastry and cook in the oven for 20 mins.

7) Serve with vegetables or salad.

Ribbon prawns and spaghetti

- 4 oz of whole wheat spaghetti
- One butternut squash
- 1 zucchini
- 2 cups of cleaned prawns
- Seasoning
- 1 cup of cherry tomatoes
- 3 cloves garlic sliced
- 1 cup of chicken stock
- Fresh chives

Method

1) Boil a pot of salted water and add spaghetti.
2) Cook as per instructions until al dente
3) Trim the top and bottom of your squash and use a vegetable peeler to create ribbons. If you have a spiralizer you can use it to create ribbons.
4) Take 60ml of the water from the pasta pot and drain the rest.
5) In a medium bowl combine the pasta and squash ribbons evenly

6) Lightly coat the prawns with seasoning and add to a frying pan on high heat.
7) Cook until just pink around the edges, approx. 2mins
8) Add tomatoes and garlic and cook until the tomatoes have softened
9) Add ribbons and stock and cook until stock reduces. Use the pasta water if the noodles seem to be drying out.
10) Season to taste and serve with chopped chives.

Grilled cauliflower with couscous

- 1 large head of cauliflower
- 2 tablespoons of harissa
- 8 tablespoons of virgin olive oil
- Salt
- 1 clove of minced garlic
- 2 tsps minced ginger
- 2 cups couscous
- 1 cup of raisins
- Lemon juice

- Cup of feta crumbled
- Half a cup of parsley
- Fresh black pepper
- 10 olives

Method

1) Turn on the grill for high-heat
2) Remove the bottom leaves of the cauliflower and slice into rounds
3) Cut each round into 4 pieces, save trimmings for later
4) Mix together harissa and 3tbsp of olive oil in a small bowl.
5) Take two pieces of foil and lay cauliflower pieces equally on them
6) Brush with harissa mixture and add salt and pepper
7) Wrap the cauliflower steaks in the foil and seal
8) Place on the grill sealed side down and cook for 10 mins
9) Flip after 10 mins and open top of the packet to allow steam to escape
10) Cook for a further 8 mins until cauliflower is tender

11) While cauliflower is cooking heat olive oil in a frying pan and add garlic and ginger
12) Add couscous, 2 cups of water and the raisins. Season to taste.
13) Bring to boil, cover and cook until the water has been absorbed, around 12 mins
14) Serve the cooked couscous along with cooked cauliflower, drizzled with lemon juice, feta, and parsley. Garnish with olives.

Maybe you need to have your lunch at work and struggle to find healthy alternatives. Here are a couple of alternatives to traditional packed lunches.

Chicken wraps

- ¾ cup of low-fat yogurt
- 2 tbsp mustard
- 1 tbsp lemon juice
- Pinch of salt
- 1 lb cooked chicken meat
- 2 oz toasted walnuts

- 6 leaves of lettuce, preferably Cos or Iceberg
- 4 whole meal wraps

Method

In a small bowl mix the yogurt, lemon juice, mustard, and seasoning together. Fold in the chicken and walnuts.

Take a lettuce leaf and place it on a wrap. Spoon around 100g of the mixture on the leaf and fold. Slice the wrap in half and serve cold.

Grilled Vegetable Panini with feta

- Mixed vegetables. Red and green peppers, zucchini or squash. Whatever your favorite grilled veg is.
- Portobello mushroom
- 4 ciabatta slices
- Olive oil for cooking and drizzling
- Seasoning
- ½ cup of crumbled feta cheese

- ½ cup of cream cheese, use flavored cheese to add taste to your panini
- 4 lettuce leaves

Method

In a grill pan grill the vegetables until tender and season to taste. Mix the feta cheese with the cream cheese and spread on ciabatta slices. Cover with the grilled veg and a lettuce leaf and return the slices to the pan. Grill until the bread is browned and the cheese is melted. Your ciabatta can now be wrapped in foil ready for your lunch.

Intermediate Level Intermittent Fasting

The 5-2 plan

This is the next level of intermittent fasting and should only be undertaken following a consult with your doctor. This plan involves eating clean for five days and fasting for the other two days. The meals you eat on your non-fasting days should be packed with healthy fats and protein to maintain your energy levels when you are fasting.

Quick tip!

If you aren't quite ready to go full on 5-2 plan you can try the modified plan. Eat clean for 5 days but restrict your calorie intake for the other two days. Aim to consume no more than 700 calories on your "fasting" days and this will help your body prepare for the 5-2 plan in its purest form.

Protein packed recipes to keep your energy levels up!

Chili Bean and Bulgur Burger

- ½ cup of bulgur wheat
- 2 tbsp virgin oil
- 4 oz tomato paste
- 1 tsp chili powder
- Black pepper
- 1/3 cup low fat soured cream
- Zest and juice of 1 lime
- Can kidney beans
- ½ cup shredded cheese
- 2 spring onions
- 1 cup of alfalfa sprouts
- Cooking spray
- 2 tbsp breadcrumbs

Method

1) Cook the bulgur wheat as per instructions and leave to cool completely
2) In a small skillet make chili oil by combining tomato paste and chili powder with virgin oil until it turns yellow

3) Mix sour cream and lime juice and zest with seasoning and place in refrigerator
4) In a blender mix the cooked bulgur, kidney beans, breadcrumbs, cheese and spring onions with seasoning.
5) Make 4 uniform patties around 3/4 of an inch thick and place onto a foil lined baking sheet.
6) Grill for 5 mins on each side until the patties are golden brown. Use cooking spray to crisp the tops.
7) Serve with avocado and alfalfa. Add sour cream lime as required.

You can make this meal more substantial with pitta bread, rolls or ciabatta to serve your burger in.

Do you love pizza but know that it is not a healthy option? Try this recipe for guilt free pizza!

Cauliflower crust pizza

- 1 medium cauliflower head
- ½ cup grated parmesan cheese
- Italian seasoning
- 2 medium eggs
- 1 Tsp salt
- 2 cups mozzarella cheese grated

Method

In a food processor pulse your cauliflower florets until they form a white powder. Take the powder and place in a bowl, cover, and microwave until soft, around 4 or 5 mins. Take the mixture and place in a clean kitchen towel and allow to cool.

When the mix is cool enough to handle grasp the kitchen towel and squeeze until you have removed as much moisture as possible. In a large bowl, combine with the rest of the ingredients. Take a baking sheet and line with parchment paper. Place the mix on the baking sheet and press into a circular shape.

Bake in a pre-heated oven at 400 degrees for 15 mins until golden. Remove from oven and you have your guilt free pizza base. Top with your favorite sauce and add your favorite toppings. Serve with a healthy salad for a filling meal.

Intermittent Fasting Hard Core, Alternative Days

Even though this plan is advanced, it is very simple! Eat every other day. Eat clean source meat, healthy fats, fruit and veg, making sure every meal is filled with energy giving stuff. On your fasting days keep hydrated with water, herbal teas, and sugar free soft drinks. A moderate amount of black tea and coffee is allowed but watch for caffeine levels.

Quick tip: If you need something to snack on when you are fasting there is a "rule" you can follow. As long as the snack is no more than 40 calories it is acceptable.

Snacks and their calorific values
Satisfy your sweet tooth
Half a small banana (40 calories)
Ten cherries (40 calories)
2 sugar-free ice pops (30 calories)

Feel like a salty snack?

8 oz miso soup (36 calories)

3 dill pickles (30 calories)

Half a cup of salty popcorn (40 calories)

Crunchy snacks

Celery stalk with natural peanut butter (40 calories)

1 brown rice cake with low fat cheese spread (40 calories)

1 small apple (35 calories)

Cheesy treats

Slice of fat free cheese (30 calories)

Large tomato with 1tbsp parmesan grilled

Rice cake with 1 oz of fat free cottage cheese

Protein power ups

1 oz of smoked salmon on a rice cake (35 calories)

2 large hardboiled egg whites with 1oz cottage cheese (40 calories)

1 water packed sardine with a slice of onion (35 calories)

Standard go-to snacks

Half a cup of melon with 1tbsp light sour cream (40 calories)

A glass of seltzer with ¼ cup of cranberry juice (33 calories)

¾ cup of almond milk (40 calories)

Power Breakfasts

The meals you do eat should be well balanced and provide you with the nutrients you require. We have covered meals that are suitable for lunch or evening meal but what should you be eating for breakfast? Here are some ideas for power breakfasts that will start your day with a healthy kick!

Berry Parfait

Combine ¼ cup of cooked quinoa, ¾ cup of low-fat yogurt, a splash of vanilla essence and a sprinkling of cinnamon. Take ¼ cup of blueberries and 6 crushed walnuts to create a layered effect with the yogurt mixture.

This tasty breakfast will give you 25 grams of protein for just over 300 calories and will keep your energy levels high.

Eggsadilla

Take one full egg and two egg whites and scramble in a pan until they are fully cooked. Place the eggs on a whole wheat tortilla and top with grated cheese and 1tbsp salsa. Roll and eat while hot.

Again 25 grams of protein for just over 300 calories. The calories can be reduced by using low fat cheese.

French toast

Take one slice of whole-grained bread and soak in a beaten egg mixture. Cook for one minute on each side in a non-stick pan, serve with ½ a cup of low-fat yogurt flavored with cinnamon.

28 grams of protein for 250 calories

Omelet

Omelets are the easiest way to add vegetables to your breakfast while increasing your protein levels.

Combine 4 egg whites with a mixture of veggies, peppers, spinach, mushrooms, tomatoes, and onion depending on your taste. Use a cooking spray to coat your frying pan and as the egg mixture starts to solidify add ½ cup of low-fat cottage cheese. Continue to cook until eggs are set, fold and serve.

28 grams protein 260 calories

Healthy scrambled eggs

This recipe is from the Mediterranean diet and is one of the healthiest ways to eat breakfast.

Combine one egg with four egg whites and scramble in a non-stick pan. Top the cooked eggs with 3tbsp light ricotta cheese and ½ cup of wilted spinach.

27 grams protein 210 calories

Spicy breakfast burrito

Scramble an egg with two egg whites and add ½ cup of pinto bean. Line a sprouted grain tortilla with avocado slices and add the egg mixture. Top with tbsp of salsa, fold and eat.

23 grams of protein 280 calories

Egg and veggie Florentine bowl

Coat an 8oz ramekin with coconut oil and add an egg, 1tbsp cold water, 2tbsp spinach, 2 chopped mushrooms and beat until blended. Microwave on high for 30 seconds and stir. Pop back into the microwave for 45 seconds until eggs are set. Remove and top with grated cheese or tomatoes.

23 grams of protein (185 calories)

Twice baked sweet potato and egg

Cook a medium sized sweet potato in the oven for 40 mins until soft. Set aside to cool. In a non-stick pan sauté 1 diced onion, ½ cup of cherry tomatoes and 2 crushed garlic cloves. When the potato is cool enough to handle scoop out the flesh from one half and combine with 4tsp of low-fat Greek yogurt, salt, and pepper and add to pan. Cook for a further 5 mins and then return to potato shell. Make a well in the center of the mixture and crack a medium egg into the well. Return to oven and cook until egg is set.

12 grams protein (206 calories)

Egg rings

Slice a large red bell pepper into ¾ inch rings and cook in a skillet for 2 mins on each side. Crack an egg into the center of the ring and cook until set. Serve with sliced avocado and a slice of gluten free bread.

15 grams of protein (200 calories)

Rainbow pinwheels

Take a whole wheat wrap and coat with pesto sauce. Add a slice of cheddar cheese and top with another whole wheat wrap. Coat the second wrap with low fat cream cheese, top with a sliced hard-boiled egg. Add a third wrap and coat with tomato sauce. Roll the wrap sandwich into a roll and slice. The colors of your ingredients will form a rainbow!

26 grams of protein (400 calories)

Fat Bombs

What are fat bombs? They are a great way to boost your levels of healthy fats. These are essential to your health and especially when you are on a fasting program. Here are a couple of tasty fat bomb recipes for you to try.

Bacon and egg fat bombs (make six servings)

2 large free-range eggs

¾ cup of melted butter

2 tbsp mayo

Seasoning

5 oz lean bacon

Method

Cook the bacon under the grill until crispy. Meanwhile, hard-boil the eggs for around 10 mins. Place cooked eggs in cold water to cool. Peel and chop the eggs and add the melted butter to the eggs. Mash with a fork, add mayo and seasoning along with any fat from the bacon. Place mixture into the fridge until chilled.

Crumble the bacon to form breading. Take the chilled mixture and form six balls using a spoon or ice cream server. Roll balls in crumbled bacon and eat as required. The fat bombs will keep for up to 5 days in an airtight container.

Sugar free peanut butter fudge

1 cup unsweetened peanut butter

1 cup coconut oil

¼ cup unsweetened almond milk

Method

1) Soften peanut butter and coconut oil in the microwave
2) Add to rest of ingredients and put in your blender
3) Blend until smooth
4) Line a baking sheet with parchment paper
5) Pour mixture onto paper

6) Refrigerate for 3 hours or overnight whenever possible

Your peanut butter fudge is now ready to eat. You can make a chocolate sauce to make it even tastier.

Combine ¼ cup of unsweetened cocoa powder with 2tbsp coconut oil and add your chosen sweetener. Drizzle over fudge before refrigerating.

Conclusion

Fasting is not a new concept when considering improving your health. History is littered with examples of fasting, but why should you try it? What do you have to lose?

Good luck on your journey to improved mental and physical health! Whatever level is comfortable for your needs, there are many stages to choose from. This book can be your first step on the ladder to healthier living. Make sure you check with your health expert before you take a rung up the ladder and stay within your comfort zone.

Fasting is not a fad, it works! Fasting can also be maintained in all walks of life. Diets have variable efficacy, fasting has been proved to be the most efficient way to lose weight and lower insulin.

Part 2

Introduction

Welcome!

If you've already started to follow the 5:2 Diet, then keep reading. If you've bought this book because you're intrigued as to what it is (Wow! A diet where I get to eat 7 meals a day! – Sorry, no...) then you might want to jump to page 3 for a short overview of the background and benefits.

As long-time followers of the 5:2 Fast Diet, we understand how easy it is to become diet-weary after a while: the same basic foods, twice a week, month after month. It's easy to hit a rut of the same low-calorie options simply in order to save effort. The initial enthusiasm in starting something new quickly wanes once the euphoria wears off and the drudgery sets in.

Finding creative and interesting options for breakfast has been especially challenging. A piece of fruit will satisfy the calorie limitations (and is a great option for rushed mornings), but what about hot breakfasts, cereals, and breads?

The key to a successful low-calorie day is preparation. If you wake up in the morning and find you have nothing in the cupboard that will give you a good-sized portion to eat without using up your entire calorie allowance, then it's going to be a struggle.

With these thoughts in mind, we set out to develop a set of 5:2-friendly breakfast recipes, including make-ahead meals, quick grab-and-go options, and even hot meat-and-potatoes dishes. We've organized the recipes into 4 sections:

Under 50 calories, for when you're saving the bulk of your fast day allotment for later in the day;

50-100 calories, for dieters who prefer 5-6 small meals or snacks throughout their fast days;

100-200 calories, for the three-squares-a-day dieter in which each meal is roughly 1/3 of the daily allotment; and

200-300 calories, for those who divide their daily calories into two main meals.

The next section gives a quick overview of the 5:2 Fast Diet and discusses meal planning strategies and survival tips in more detail. We've also included charts of common fruits and other breakfast-friendly foods that list the calories per gram, along with typical portion sizes.

A note about ingredients: What you won't find in any of these recipes are artificial sweeteners and other such "diet" foods. We believe that the 5:2 is a lifelong eating plan, not a lose-weight-fast scheme, and as such, needs to be sustainable and healthy in the long term. Without commenting on the conflicting and sometimes acrimonious research as to the long-term effects of artificial sweeteners, we prefer to err on the side of caution and focus on healthy, natural alternatives.

Overview of The 5:2 Fast Diet

The 5:2 Diet (also written as 5+2) is an eating plan based on the concept of **Intermittent Fasting** (IF). As the name implies, IF alternates higher calorie days with lower calorie days, the theory being that these caloric swings trigger the body to produce an abundance of beneficial chemicals. Because the chemicals that are released are thought to forestall medical disorders often associated with aging such as adult onset diabetes and dementia, IF has been touted for years as an anti-aging diet.

The 5:2 Diet uses the basic principles of IF – high and low calorie days – but adds a bit more structure in order to make the diet plan easier to follow. Note here that "high" calorie means the normal recommended intake. This isn't a binge-and-bust diet, and in fact you're more likely to discover that on non-fast days you'll be more aware of how many calories you're eating and will scale back compared to your habits before trying the diet.

It's not a weight loss diet *per se*, but most people who follow the diet find that they lose some weight, and that it stays lost. We'll come back to this shortly.

How it works

The 5:2 Diet is one of the simplest eating plans to follow that we've come across. No food lists, no points, no exercise requirements. Simply choose two days in your week to be your "fast days" and on these days only, restrict your total calories to 500 for women, 600 for men. For the rest of the week you can eat whatever you'd like (well, almost). That's basically it! A few finer points:

1. The fast days can be done over any 24-hour time period. So instead of a traditional day, you can distribute your 500/600 calories from noon to noon, or 6 PM to 6 PM, or whatever works best for your schedule. For example, you could have a regular breakfast and

lunch (say done by 12:30), followed by a light dinner and a light breakfast the next morning, then back to a regular lunch (after 12:30 the next day).

That said, we've found from personal experience that we "feel" more benefit from the diet by sticking to a single day, probably because that extends the fast time by having a block of sleep at either end.

2. Dr. Michael Mosley, pioneer of the 5:2 and author of *The Fast Diet*, recommends that the two fast days not be done back-to-back. They should be separated by at least a day, presumably to prevent the body from going into hunger mode from prolonged calorie reductions.

3. If you require a high calorie intake, because of regular exercise or a manual job, then you may need to increase your calorie allotment on the fast days. On the other hand, if you're of slight build, then you may find that you can go lower than the recommended

500/600: some people even go to the extreme of two zero-calorie days per week.

Does it work?

The two main benefits touted by IF are improved health and weight loss. Here's a summary of the medical evidence for each.

Improved health: Most of the formal medical studies on IF are based on animal testing, which aren't necessarily conclusive for humans. A study by the National Institute of Aging reportedly linked IF with lower levels of IGF-1, a biomarker associated with Alzheimer's and Parkinson's diseases, but the results are difficult to assess. Other agencies, such as the UK's National Health Service, outright dismiss health benefits of IF and strongly suggest the diet be avoided.

Formal medical studies aside, however, there's plenty of anecdotal evidence – personal testimonies and informal studies – that suggests the 5:2 can help lower the risk of cancer and heart disease, and increase overall energy. Dr Mosley tracked his cholesterol and blood sugar levels while following the 5:2, and measured significant decreases in both after only just nine weeks.

Weight loss: This one's a bit tricky. If you keep your calories on the non-fast days to "normal" levels – approximately 2000 for women and 2400 for men – you *will* lose weight. The math is simple: your weekly calorie deficit from IF is about 3000 for women, 3600 for men. Since every 3500 calories saved equates to one pound of weight loss, this means that men can expect to drop about a pound a week, women slightly less (about 85% of a pound, or about 6 pounds every 7 weeks). However, this does assume that you were at a stable weight to start with, and not slowly adding the pounds.

Adding just a bit of light exercise can help speed up the weight loss. For instance a moderately-paced 30 minute walk burns about 100 calories. Doing this three times per week will bump female dieters just about to the one pound/week mark.

On the other hand, overeating on the non-fast days can reduce your weight loss to nothing. You'll still get the health benefits and the anti-aging boost, but your waistline won't budge.

Survival Tips

The 5:2 Diet is one of the easiest plans to follow, but there are things you can do to make it even easier:

You don't need to commit to the same two fast days each week. Look over your schedule for the week ahead and **choose the two days that make the most sense**. Just make sure to leave a 24-hour block of non-fast time in between.

Drink plenty of water on fast days – 8-10 glasses – to stave off both hunger and dehydration. Clear broth, miso soup, and coffee/tea can also help, but be sure to include the calories, particularly the milk if you take it in coffee or tea. Look for low sodium products to prevent bloating.

It might take a few trials to ***come up with a fast day calorie distribution*** that works for your body. Some people prefer to eat a light breakfast (~200 calories) and a light dinner, and skip lunch altogether. Others eat a mid-afternoon lunch and skip dinner. What works for me personally is a 100 calorie breakfast, 150 calorie lunch, 100 calorie afternoon snack, and a 150 calorie dinner. I also reserve about 10 calories for sipping on chicken or veggie broth after work. Read more about calorie distributions in the next section.

Focus on vegetables and lean protein on your fast days to feel fuller and sustain your energy. A couple of low-cal cookies might fit the calories requirements, but could swing you toward an energy low. I like veggie-egg white frittata, vegetable soups (made with broth, not milk or cream), and salads with tuna, ham, salmon, etc. They provide a full meal but at much lower calories.

Advance planning of your fast-day meals can help to shift your focus away from food and hunger. I try to sketch out the entire day's food plan the night before to ensure that my calories will be distributed throughout the day and that I'm getting a balanced assortment of foods. Planning ahead of time can also help to make each small meal is as filling as possible.

Using weights to calculate calories instead of volume for many fruits and vegetables can help to ensure accurate calorie counts. You can pack way more sliced mushrooms or sliced strawberries into a one-cup measure than leaving them whole, right? Simply looking up the calories per cup, unless you specify whole or sliced, is either going to put you over your limit or leave you shortchanged. We recommend using an inexpensive food scale to weigh everything, then using the weight to determine the calories.

Kicking up the seasoning level on fast days really seems to trick your brain into finding the smaller meals more satisfying than they probably are. The calories in the seasoning still have to be counted, but they're usually minimal, around 5 or so per teaspoon. I find spicy and zesty blends can really help, such as fajita seasoning on chicken, creole seasoning on eggs, and sriracha on vegetables.

Meal Planning Strategies

Regardless of how you distribute your calories, it's important to mix up the types of foods that are giving you your calories.

For **breakfast**, mixing in a small amount of cereal with your fruit will give slow-release sugars to see you through the morning. Cereals tend to be high in calories (up to 4 per gram) so go easy, and use fat-free milk if you must have some. You can even get away with a small amount of lean, grilled bacon if you plan for it.

At **lunch**, go for calorie-efficient protein foods like tuna and chicken white meat (1.1 and 1.7 calories per gram). Match with a salad, leave the oil out of the dressing and stick to vinegar, and if it's going to be your main meal add a small amount of rice, potatoes or couscous if you need the carbohydrates.

Dinner is then the easy one, where you use up the remaining calories for the day. But don't forget the point of the diet is to restrict your intake, so eat what you need to and don't feel you have to go all the way to the limit if you can manage without.

5:2 Diet Power Foods

No matter how you assign the calories during the day the key to 5:2 fasting is to choose foods have a low "caloric density;" that is, foods with a low calorie content per gram. In practice this means primarily fruits, vegetables, fat-free dairy, and lean meat or fish. Oily foods including butter and so on, and foods high in carbohydrates like rice, pasta, and bread, are best used in moderation or saved for non-fasting days.

For breakfast, if you don't have the time to prepare a meal, fruit can be a great grab-and-go option. To make your calories go further, look for fruits with calorie contents of 1 calorie per gram or less. See the table below for some great breakfast choices:

Fruit	Calories Per Gram	Typical Serving Size	Calories per Serving
Star fruit	.31	1 medium (91 g)	28
Strawberries	.33	1 cup (144 g)	47
Cantaloupe	.34	1 cup (160 g)	54
Peach	.39	1 medium (150 g)	59
Watermelon	.40	1 cup (152 g)	46
Grapefruit	.42	½ medium (123	52

		g)	
Blackberries	.43	1 cup (144 g)	62
Papaya	.43	1 small (157 g)	67
Plum	.46	1 medium (66 g)	30
Orange	.47	1 medium (131 g)	62
Apricot	.48	2 medium (70 g)	34
Cherries	.50	1 cup, with pits (103 g)	51
Pineapple	.50	1 cup (165 g)	82

Apple	.52	1 medium (182 g)	95
Raspberries	.53	1 cup (123 g)	65
Blueberries	.57	1 cup (148 g)	85
Pear	.57	1 medium (178 g)	102
Mango *	.60	1 cup (165 g)	99
Kiwi	.61	1 medium (69 g)	42
Guava	.68	1 cup (165 g)	112
Grapes *	.69	1 cup (151 g)	104
Banana *	.89	1	105

		medium (118 g)	
Passion Fruit *	.97	2 fruits (36 g)	34

* These fruits tend to be higher in sugar – more than 10% by weight – so alternate with other fruits for lasting energy throughout the morning.

In addition to fruits, many vegetables and lean proteins also have reasonably low caloric densities. Some of the more breakfast-friendly options (for omelets and quiche, for example) are shown in the table below. We've also included some lower calorie carbs for the days when you need a heartier breakfast. Stock up on these and you'll always have ingredients on hand for fast days.

Food	Calories Per Gram	Typical Serving Size	Calories per Serving
Mushrooms (raw)	.16	½ cup (113 g)	18
Asparagus (cooked)	.22	1 cup (90 g)	20
Spinach (raw)	.23	1 cup (30 g)	7
Broccoli (cooked)	.28	½ cup (92 g)	26
Artichoke	.30	½ cup	34

Hearts		(113 g)	
Tomato	.30	1 medium (91 g)	16
Bell pepper	.30	½ medium (60 g)	12
Egg white	.48	1 large (33 g)	16
Fat-free milk	.42	½ cup (122 g)	51
Fat-free plain yogurt	.47	4 oz. (113 g)	53
Oatmeal (cooked)	.71	½ cup (117 g)	83
Potato	.75	½ medium (87 g)	65
Black beans (cooked)	.91	½ cup (121 g)	110
Brown rice (cooked)	1.03	½ cup (97 g)	100

Fat-free feta	1.07	2 oz. (56 g)	60
Smoked salmon	1.16	2 oz. (28 g)	66

Recipes: Under 50 Calories Per Serving

It's not easy to put together a filling meal for fewer than 50 calories per serving. But for those days when you need to save the bulk of your calories for later in the day, these small meals can be a lifesaver. To get the most food for the fewest calories, we've focused on ingredients that have very low calories per gram, such as fruits and fish.

Mixed Fruit Salad (49 calories)

Baked Pear (44 calories)

Broiled Tomato (49 calories)

Berry Parfait (48 calories)

Smoked Salmon and Tomato (49 calories)

Veggie Frittata (47 calories)

Mixed Fruit Salad

Mix up a batch of salad the night before your fast day and separate into individual servings – you'll have a ready-to-eat option for breakfast or lunch.

Number of servings:	Serving size:	Calories per serving
4	¾ cup (125 g)	49

1 cup cantaloupe or other melon, cubed *(54 calories)*

1 cup watermelon, cubed *(46 calories)*

½ cup strawberries, sliced *(24 calories)*

⅓ cup pineapple, cubed *(27 calories)*

¼ cup blueberries *(22 calories)*

¼ cup raspberries *(16 calories)*

Instructions:

1. If you plan to prepare this ahead of time and eat throughout the week, mix

only the cantaloupe and pineapple. Cover and refrigerate.
2. On your fast days, add in the watermelon, strawberries, blueberries, and raspberries. This will help to keep the softer fruits from breaking down.

Preparation Notes:

Most blends of fruits work well. To get the most filling mix, use larger quantities of lower calorie fruits (strawberries, cantaloupe, watermelon, etc.) and supplement with a few pieces of higher calorie options. See the <u>table</u> in Chapter 2 for suggestions.

Although we've listed the ingredients with volume measurements, your calorie counts will be more accurate if you measure by weight.

Per Serving:

Calories	Fat	Carbohydrates	Protein	Sodium
49	0	11 g	1 g	7 mg

Baked Pear

For a very low-calorie breakfast or to add a bit of sweetness to your meal, try a pear baked with cinnamon, lemon, and a tart preserve.

Number of servings:	Serving size:	Calories per serving
2	½ pear	44

1 small pear

1 tsp. tart jam, such as lingonberry

½ tsp. cinnamon

1 tsp. lemon juice

½ tsp. brown sugar

Cooking spray

Instructions:

1. *Preheat oven to 350 F.*
2. Spray a small baking dish with cooking spray.
3. Cut the pear in half and scoop out the seeds and core, leaving a small well in

the center of each half. Place in baking dish (cut side up).
4. Sprinkle ½ tsp. of lemon juice onto each pear half, top with cinnamon, then sprinkle with the brown sugar.
5. Put ½ tsp. of jam into each of the scooped-out wells.
6. Place the baking pan into the oven and bake for about 20 minutes until tender.

Preparation Notes:

If using a sweeter jam, omit the brown sugar. (The calories work out to be about the same.)

Per Serving:

Calories	Fat	Carbohydrates	Protein	Sodium
44	0 g	13 g	0 g	1 mg

Broiled Tomato

Tomatoes are a 5:2 dieter's best friend! Low in calories and packed with nutrients, this recipe is great on its own or as an accompaniment to a larger meal.

Number of servings:	Serving size:	Calories per serving
2	½ tomato	49

1 large tomato
1 tsp. dijonnaise spread***
1 Tbsp. shredded mozzarella cheese
1 Tbsp. panko or other coarse bread crumbs
1 tsp. parmesan cheese
Cooking spray

Instructions:

1. *Preheat the broiler.*
2. Coat a small baking tray with cooking spray.
3. Slice the tomato in half and place into the tray. Spread ½ tsp. of dijonnaise onto each half.
4. Mix the mozzarella and panko crumbs together, and press onto the tomato halves.
5. Broil for about 1 minute then turn off the oven. Tent a sheet of aluminum foil

over the tomatoes and leave in the hot oven until cooked through, about 5-10 minutes.
6. Remove from the oven and sprinkle ½ tsp. parmesan onto each half.

Preparation Notes:

*** If you don't have prepared dijonnaise spread, make your own by combining ½ tsp. of light mayonnaise with 2-½ tsp. Dijon mustard (makes 1 Tbsp. of spread).

For an even lower calorie meal, omit the mozzarella and season the breadcrumbs with a few shakes of Italian seasoning. Lightly spray with cooking spray before broiling. Made this way you'll shave off about 10 calories per serving.

Per Serving:

Calories	Fa	Carbohydrates	Protein	Sodium
49	1.	7 g	2.5 g	106 mg

Berry Parfait

Super quick, low calorie breakfast with fresh fruit and high-protein Greek yogurt.

Number of servings:	Serving size:	Calories per serving
1	1 portion	48

¼ cup strawberries, sliced

¼ cup raspberries

2 Tbsp. plain Greek yogurt, fat-free

1 tsp. <u>low fat granola</u>

Instructions:

1. *Mix the strawberries and raspberries together in a bowl.*
2. Add the fruit to a small glass and top with the yogurt.
3. Sprinkle with granola.

Preparation Notes:

Most combinations of berries work well in this recipe. Use the <u>table</u> in Chapter 2 to make sure the fruit calories don't exceed 30.

Per Serving:

Calories	Fat	Carbohydrates	Protein	Sodium
49	0 g	8.5 g	2.5 g	12 mg

Smoked Salmon and Tomatoes

Protein-packed fish and nutrient-rich tomatoes make a perfect start to the day.

Number of servings:	Serving size:	Calories per serving
1	1 portion	49

1 ounce (28 grams) smoked salmon
1 medium tomato, very ripe
½ Tbsp. capers

Instructions:

1. Slice the tomato into thin sections and arrange on a plate.

2. Slice the salmon into strips and distribute evenly onto the tomato slices.
3. Coarsely chop the capers and sprinkle on top of the salmon.

Preparation Notes:

The calories in smoked salmon can vary widely, so read the labels carefully. In general, wild-caught salmon is less fatty than farm-raised, so the calories will be lower. This recipe uses salmon with 35 calories per ounce (1.25 calories per gram).

Capers are a great addition to the 5:2 Diet. With only 5 calories per tablespoon, they pack an enormous amount of flavor for very few calories.

Per serving:

Calories	Fat	Carbohydrates	Protein	Sodium
49	1.5	5 g	6.5 g	700 mg

Veggie Frittata

Two egg whites, a splash of milk, and a ton of veggies make for a power breakfast on your low-calorie fast days.

Number of servings:	Serving size:	Calories per serving
1	1 portion	47

2 egg whites

½ cup fresh spinach leaves, chopped

¼ red bell pepper, chopped

1 Tbsp. fat-free milk

Spray oil

Instructions:

1. *Preheat oven to 350 F.*
2. Spray a small ovenproof skillet with oil. Add the bell pepper and cook over low heat until cooked through.
3. Stir the spinach into the pepper and cook until the leaves are wilted, about 30 seconds.

4. While the vegetables are cooking, whisk together the egg whites and milk.
5. Pour the egg mixture over the vegetables and stir.
6. Move the skillet to the oven and bake for 8-10 minutes or until set.

Preparation Notes:

Any of the vegetables from the table in Chapter 2 (5:2 Diet Power Foods) will work well in this recipe. Be sure to adjust the calories accordingly.

Per serving:

Calories	Fat	Carbohydrates	Protein	Sodium
47	0 g	3.5 g	8.5 g	124 mg

Recipes: 50-100 Calories Per Serving

If you need a bigger meal to kick-start to the day, try one of these recipes. They all include a dose of carbohydrates or protein that will make you feel fuller for longer.

<u>Whole Wheat Blueberry Muffins</u> (93 calories)

<u>Veggie-Sausage Spinach Cups</u> (91 calories)

<u>Low-Calorie Strawberry Granola</u> (78 calories)

<u>Chicken-Apple Sausage Patties</u> (89 calories)

<u>Multi-Grain English Muffins</u> (97 calories)

<u>Orange Juice Cranberry Muffins</u> (94 calories)

Whole Wheat Blueberry Muffins

Made with whole grain, fruit, and protein-packed Greek yogurt, these muffins are a great fast day choice for breakfast on the go. Make in advance and store in the freezer for a quick and filling 100-calorie meal.

Number of servings:	Serving size:	Calories per serving
6 muffins	1 muffin (60 g)	93

¾ cup whole wheat flour

1 tsp. baking powder

¼ tsp. salt

1 egg white

½ cup plain Greek yogurt, fat-free

⅛cup brown sugar

1 Tbsp. applesauce, unsweetened

1 cup blueberries, fresh or frozen (thawed)

Baking spray

Instructions:

1. Preheat oven to 375 F.

2. Coat six standard-size muffin cups with baking spray or spray oil.
3. In a medium mixing bowl, stir together the flour, baking powder, and salt.
4. In a separate bowl, whisk together the egg white, yogurt, brown sugar, and applesauce.
5. Slowly pour the liquid mixture into the flour mixture, stirring lightly until just mixed. Gently stir in the blueberries.
6. Spoon the batter into the 6 prepared muffin cups, dividing equally. Don't fill to more than about 2/3.
7. Bake in the preheated oven about 15 minutes or until golden. The tops should spring back when pressed lightly.
8. Allow muffins to cool in the pan 5 minutes, then transfer onto a wire rack and cool completely.

Preparation Notes:

The whole wheat flour can make these a bit denser than muffins made with white flour. To keep them fluffy, do not over stir the batter in Step 5.

Per Muffin:

Calories	Fat	Carbohydrates	Protein	Sodium
93	0.5	19.5 g	3.5 g	112 mg

Veggie-Sausage Spinach Cups

The protein in these tasty breakfast casserole cups will sustain you all morning. They'll keep for a couple of days in the refrigerator and a month or so in the freezer.

Number of servings:	Serving size:	Calories per serving
4	1 muffin (132 g)	91

3 oz. fresh spinach

2 eggs

2 egg whites

⅛ cup fat-free milk

2 oz. crumbled veggie sausage

2 oz. shredded mozzarella cheese

Spray oil

Salt & pepper

Instructions:

1. *Preheat oven to 375 F.*
2. Coat four standard-size muffin cups with cooking spray.
3. Lightly coat a non-stick skillet with cooking spray and heat to medium-low. Add the spinach and sauté until just soft, adding a teaspoon of water if the spinach starts to stick.
4. While the spinach is cooking, whisk together in a small bowl the eggs, egg whites, and milk.
5. When the spinach has cooked, divide into six portions and place into the prepared muffin cups.
6. In each cup, top the spinach with a spoonful of veggie sausage.
7. Pour the egg mixture into each cup, filling about 2/3 full.

8. Top each cup with a pinch of shredded cheese and sprinkle with salt and pepper.
9. Bake the casserole cups for about 15 minutes.

Preparation Notes:

If you don't care for veggie sausage, you can substitute turkey sausage patties or <u>chicken-apple sausage</u> (broken up into crumbles). This adds 10 calories per serving to the recipe.

Per Muffin:

Calories	Fat	Carbohydrates	Protein	Sodium
91	5.5	2 g	9 g	200 mg

Low-Calorie Strawberry Granola

Most commercially-prepared granolas are packed with calories. To lighten up, we've left out the nuts and most of the fat, and sweetened with agave nectar for sustained energy.

Number of servings:	Serving size:	Calories per serving
4	1 muffin (132 g)	91

2 cups old-fashioned oats

½ cup wheat germ

2 cups dried strawberries

¼ cup agave nectar

3 Tbsp. flaxseed oil

1 tsp. vanilla extract

1 Tbsp. water

Spray oil

Instructions:

1. *Preheat oven to 275 F.*
2. In a medium mixing bowl, stir together the oats and wheat germ.
3. In a small sauce pan, heat the agave nectar, flaxseed oil, vanilla extract, and water over low heat. Bring to a simmer but do not boil.
4. Pour the liquid over the oat mixture and stir thoroughly.

5. Coat a large baking tray with spray oil and add the oat mixture, spreading evenly.
6. Bake for 30 minutes, then stir in the strawberries. Spread the granola evenly in the tray and continue to bake for another 15 minutes.

Preparation Notes:

You can substitute honey for the agave nectar (thin with a little water) without changing the calories.

Other dried fruits work well, too. For a variation try:

Dried *cherries* (unsweetened): Reduce the quantity to a scant 1 cup. The calories per serving increase to 100.

Dried *blueberries*: Use the full 2 cups. The calories per serving increases to 82.

Dried *cranberries* (unsweetened): Use the full 2 cups. The calories per serving don't change.

Per Serving:

Calories	Fat	Carbohydrates	Protein	Sodium
78	3 g	11.5 g	2 g	0 mg

Chicken-Apple Sausage Patties

Although sausage isn't always the healthiest breakfast choice, these patties break the rule! Made with lean chicken breast and farm-fresh apples, these are great on their own or paired with an <u>egg or potatoes</u> (when you've got more calories to spare).

Number of servings:	Serving size:	Calories per serving
8	2 patties (83 g)	89

2 tsp. canola oil

1 medium apple, peeled and diced

1 lb. ground chicken breast

1 tsp. dried sage

1 Tbsp. light brown sugar

½ tsp. fennel seed, ground

¾ tsp. salt

¼ tsp. black pepper

Spray oil

Instructions:

1. *Heat the canola oil over medium heat in a nonstick skillet. Add the diced apples and cook for two minutes. Move the apples to a bowl for cooling.*
2. In a medium mixing bowl, combine the chicken, sage, sugar, fennel seed, salt, and pepper. Mix well to a uniform consistency, then stir in the cooked apples.
3. Divide the meat mixture into 16 equal portions. Form each portion into a ball, then press gently to form a 3-inch patty.
4. Spray the skillet with cooking spray and heat over low. Cook the patties (three or four at a time) for 3 minutes on each side, or until browned and cooked through. If the outsides are cooking too quickly, add a small amount of water to the pan and cover.

Preparation Notes:

I typically make these with a sweeter apple such as Gala or Honeycrisp. But for a different taste, try one that's more tart, such as Granny Smith or McIntosh.

Per Serving:

Calories	Fat	Carbohydrates	Protein	Sodium
89	1.5	4.5 g	14 g	250 mg

Multi-Grain English Muffins

Skip the store-bought "100-calorie" muffins, they're often laden with artificial sweeteners. This recipe comes in at the same calorie content, but with all-natural ingredients. These take some time for the yeast to rise, so make ahead for a morning treat.

Number of servings:	Serving size:	Calories per serving
13	1 muffin (46 g)	97

½ cup warm water

1 Tbsp. agave nectar or honey

2 tsp. yeast (active dry)

1 tsp. butter, melted

1-½ cups all-purpose flour

1 cup whole wheat flour

¼ cup rolled oats

¼ cup wheat germ

1 Tbsp. salt

2 tsp. whole flaxseed

½ cup low-fat or fat-free buttermilk

Cooking spray

Instructions:

1. *In a small cup, stir the agave nectar (or honey) and yeast into the water and allow the mixture to froth. Stir in the melted butter.*
2. Using a large mixing bowl, combine the flours, oats, wheat germ, salt, and flaxseed. Add the buttermilk and yeast mixture and form into dough with your hands.

3. Dust your work surface with flour and turn out the dough. Knead for about 4 minutes until smooth.
4. Spray a mixing bowl with oil and place the dough into the bowl. Cover the bowl with a cloth towel and put in a warm location to rise, about an hour. The dough should double in size.
5. When the dough is ready, knead for another 2 minutes on a lightly floured work surface. Roll into a sheet about ½-inch thick.
6. Use a round biscuit or cookie cutter (3-inch diameter) to cut out the muffins. Place the rounds on a cookie sheet (line with parchment paper or use a silicone baking sheet), cover with a cloth, and allow to rise for 20 minutes until puffy.
7. Spray a large skillet or griddle with cooking spray and heat to low. Add a few of the rounds, keeping them about 2 inches apart. Cook about 5-6 minutes per side or until golden. Repeat for the remainder of the dough. Allow the muffins to cool for about 20 minutes before splitting.

Per Serving:

Calories	Fat	Carbohydrates	Protein	Sodium
97	1	18.5 g	3 g	550 mg

Orange Juice Cranberry Muffins

While not the lowest calorie-per-gram option, sometimes you just need a muffin! These healthy alternatives freeze well, too – make in advance and enjoy throughout the week.

Number of servings:	Serving size:	Calories per serving
12	1 muffin (49 g)	94

2 cups all-purpose flour
2 tsp. baking powder
1 Tbsp. orange zest
1 egg
¾ cup orange juice
¼ cup applesauce
2 Tbsp. milk
1 tsp. vanilla

½ cup dried cranberries, chopped

Baking spray

Instructions:

1. *Preheat oven to 400 F.*
2. In a large mixing bowl, combine the flour, baking powder, and orange zest.
3. Stir in the egg, orange juice, applesauce, milk, and vanilla. Mix lightly until just blended. The batter will be a bit lumpy, but don't over mix.
4. Stir in the cranberries.
5. Coat 12 muffin cups with baking spray and fill each about half full with batter.
6. Bake 8-12 minutes until just browned. The tops should spring back when pressed lightly.
7. Cool the muffins in the pan for about 5 minutes then move to a cooling rack. Let cool on the rack for another 5-10 minutes before serving.

Preparation Notes:

Stir the wet ingredients into the flour mixture until just wet. Over mixing can make the muffins too dense.

Per Muffin:

Calories	Fat	Carbohydrates	Protein	Sodium
90	0.5	19.5 g	3 g	8 mg

Recipes: 100-200 Calories Per Serving

These recipes give you a bigger calorie boost, so that the start of your fast day isn't such a shock. Go for these if you need the extra energy to see you through to the afternoon.

Potato-Ham Frittata (118 calories)

Smoked Salmon Breakfast Sandwich (168 calories)

Breakfast Bread Pudding (125 calories)

Apple Crisp (135 calories)

Huevos Rancheros (169 calories)

Fish Fingers (165 calories)

Classic American Breakfast: Bacon, Eggs, and Hash Browns (175 calories)

Mini Hash Brown Casseroles (149 calories)

Potato-Ham Frittata

When you're craving an old-school meat-and-potatoes breakfast or brunch, try this low-calorie frittata. When made with egg substitute, it's low in fat, too, and packed with protein.

Number of servings:	Serving size:	Calories per serving
4	1 portion (164 g)	118

1-½ cups egg substitute
2 Tbsp. fat-free milk
1/4 tsp. salt
Pinch of thyme
Pinch of black pepper
¼ cup chopped green pepper
2 cups shredded potato (raw)
½ cup chopped ham
1 Tbsp. cheddar cheese, grated

Spray oil

Instructions:

1. *Place the shredded potatoes in a microwave-safe bowl and microwave for 2 minutes.*

2. In a separate bowl, beat together the eggs, milk, salt, thyme, and black pepper.
3. Coat a medium skillet with spray oil and cook the green pepper until tender, about 2 minutes. Add the potatoes and continue cooking for about 5 minutes until the potatoes are lightly browned.
4. Stir in the ham and cook for another minute.
5. Pour the egg mixture into the skillet and cover. Cook for about 8 minutes, occasionally lifting the edges of the frittata so that the uncooked egg flows to the bottom.
6. When the frittata has set, sprinkle with cheese. Cover the skillet and heat until the cheese is just melted, about 30 seconds.
7. Remove from heat, cut into 4 servings, and serve.

Preparation Notes:

If you prefer, replace the egg substitute with 6 large eggs. The calories per serving will increase to 162.

Per Serving:

Calories	Fat	Carbohydrates	Protein	Sodium
118	2 g	8.5 g	15.5 g	565 mg

Smoked Salmon Breakfast Sandwich

A healthy alterative to a traditional breakfast, this lower calorie version is made with egg whites and salmon on a multi-grain muffin.

Number of servings:	Serving size:	Calories per serving
1	1 sandwich (169 g)	168

2 egg whites

Pinch of salt

1 tsp. capers

1 ounce smoked salmon

2 slices of tomato

1 <u>low-calorie multi-grain English muffin</u>, split and toasted

Spray oil

Instructions:

1. *Spray a small skillet with oil and heat over medium heat.*
2. Rinse the capers and chop coarsely.
3. Add the egg whites, salt, and capers to the frying pan. Cook while stirring constantly for about 30 seconds or until the egg whites are set.
4. Put one half of the muffin onto a plate and top with the egg whites. Top with the smoked salmon and the tomato slice, and cover with the other muffin half.

Preparation Notes:

For more texture and flavor, chop additional tomato and mix in with the egg white before cooking. Add about 5 calories to the total.

If you prefer, replace the egg white with 1 large egg. Total calories per serving will increase to 199.

Smoked salmon can vary widely in calories. Look for wild rather than farm-raised, and avoid the flavored varieties.

This recipe uses Scottish salmon with about 35 calories per ounce (1.25 calories per gram).

Per Serving:

Calories	Fat	Carbohydrates	Protein	Sodium
168	2.5	27 g	17.5 g	1077 mg

Breakfast Bread Pudding

Kick start your morning with a hot, baked breakfast the whole family will enjoy. The milk and egg whites start you off with a protein burst, while the whole wheat adds slow-release energy for lasting fullness.

Number of servings:	Serving size:	Calories per serving
8	1 portion (129 g)	125

6 slices low-fat, whole wheat bread

2 Tbsp. applesauce

8 egg whites

2 cups fat-free milk

¼ cup raisins

¼ cup brown sugar

1 tsp. ground cinnamon

1 tsp. vanilla extract

Baking spray

Instructions:

1. *Preheat oven to 350 F.*
2. Coat an 8 x 8 glass baking dish with baking spray or spray oil.
3. Tear bread into 1 inch pieces and place into the baking dish.
4. In a medium mixing bowl, whisk together the applesauce, egg whites, and milk. Stir in the raisins, sugar, cinnamon, and vanilla.
5. Pour the liquid mixture over the bread. Use a fork to gently press down on the bread so that it absorbs the liquid.
6. Bake in the preheated oven for 45 minutes until lightly browned. The top should spring back when pressed lightly.
7. Allow to cool for about 5 minutes before slicing.

Preparation Notes:

The calories in bread can vary widely. This recipe uses whole wheat bread with about 70 calories per 1 ounce slice (2.5 calories per gram).

For a different flavor, replace the raisins with dried cherries and add 1 additional tablespoon of brown sugar to offset the tartness. The total calories per serving will increase to 130.

Per Serving:

Calories	Fat	Carbohydrates	Protein	Sodium
125	1 g	21 g	8.5 g	200 mg

Apple Crisp

Warm cinnamon apples topped with whipped lemon yogurt is a perfect fall breakfast. This recipe scales down nicely for a single serving.

Number of servings:	Serving size:	Calories per serving
4	1 portion (115 g)	135

1 Tbsp. coconut oil

2 medium apples, cored and sliced thin

1 Tbsp. brown sugar

¼ tsp. ground ginger

Dash ground cinnamon

2 Tbsp. plain Greek yogurt, fat-free

1 tsp. grated lemon peel

4 tsp. agave nectar

¼ cup <u>low-fat granola</u>

Instructions:

1. *Melt the coconut oil over medium heat in a non-stick skillet.*
2. Add the apple slices and cook for 3 minutes.
3. Stir in the sugar, ginger, and cinnamon and continue cooking until the apples are cooked through.
4. While the apples are cooking, whip the lemon peel into the yogurt until light and fluffy.
5. When the apples are done, divide into 4 servings and place onto plates or in shallow bowls.
6. Top each plate with ½ Tbsp. of the whipped yogurt, followed by 1 tsp. of agave nectar. Sprinkle with the granola and enjoy.

Preparation Notes:

While any type of apples will work in this recipe, crisper varieties tend to hold up the best. Look for Gala or Honeycrisp. The calories in this recipe are based on medium apples with about 182 g each.

If you prefer honey instead of agave nectar, use the same amount (1 tsp. per serving) and add 5 calories.

You can also cook the apples using butter or canola oil for about the same calories per serving.

Per Serving:

Calories	Fat	Carbohydrates	Protein	Sodium
135	3 g	26 g	1 g	50 mg

Huevos Rancheros

Living in California during college, I grew to love a big plate of huevos rancheros in the morning. While this 5:2-friendly version takes a few liberties, the tradeoff is a breakfast meal significantly lower in both fat and calories.

Number of servings:	Serving size:	Calories per serving
1	1 portion (165 g)	169

1 6-inch corn tortilla

1 egg

¼ cup fat-free refried beans

2 Tbsp. salsa

Spray oil

Instructions:

1. *Spray a medium skillet with oil and cook the tortilla on each side until heated through.*
2. Remove the tortilla from the skillet, add another spray of oil, and fry the egg until the white is set. *[Typically, huevos rancheros are served with the yolk slightly runny; however consuming undercooked eggs may increase your risk of foodborne illness, especially if you have certain medical conditions.]*
3. In a small microwave-safe bowl, cook the beans for 1 minute, stirring halfway through.
4. Place the tortilla on a plate and spread with the beans. Top with the egg and drizzle with salsa.

Preparation Notes:

The calories in this recipe are based on a 52-calorie tortilla.

For a different take on this classic dish, substitute ¼ cup cooked black beans for the refried beans (add 10 calories).

You'll save about 30 calories by replacing the egg with 2 egg whites. Mix in a little of the salsa while cooking to add flavor.

Per Serving:

Calories	Fat	Carbohydrates	Protein	Sodium
169	5 g	21 g	11 g	550 mg

Fish Fingers

For a change from traditional breakfast foods, try fish fingers with a dab of ketchup and a small handful of crackers. The protein and slow-release carbs will get you through to lunch.

Number of servings:	Serving size:	Calories per serving
3	3 fish sticks (85 g)	165

4 oz. mild white fish, such as cod or flounder

Salt & pepper

¼ cup all-purpose flour

1 egg

1 egg white

1 tsp. lemon juice

¼ cup breadcrumbs

Pinch of paprika

Cooking spray

Instructions:

1. *Preheat oven to 400 F.*
2. Spray a baking sheet with cooking spray.
3. Slice the fish into 9 approximately equally-sized strips and season lightly with salt and pepper.
4. Pour the flour into a bowl.
5. In a second bowl, whisk together the egg, egg white, and lemon juice.
6. In a third bowl, mix breadcrumbs and paprika.
7. One at a time, roll each strip of fish in flour, then coat with the egg mixture. Roll in the breadcrumbs and place on the baking tray. Continue until all strips are coated.
8. Bake in the pre-heated oven for 15 minutes, turning halfway through.

Preparation Notes:

To complete your meal add a few low-calorie crackers (about 11 g) and a side of ketchup. This adds about 45 calories.

For an even simpler breakfast, use prepared frozen fish sticks and cook per the package instructions. Look for fish sticks that are low in calories and fat.

Per Serving:

Calories	Fat	Carbohydrates	Protein	Sodium
165	5 g	15 g	14.5 g	85 mg

Classic American Breakfast: Bacon, Eggs, and Hash Browns

Craving traditional bacon and eggs for your morning meal? Try this low-calorie recipe with all the flavor but fewer than 200 calories per serving.

Number of servings:	Serving size:	Calories per serving
1	1 portion	175

1 egg

3 strips center cut bacon

½ medium potato

Cooking spray

Instructions:

1. *Preheat oven to 400°F.*
2. Using a food processor or grater, shred the potato into narrow strips. Place into a microwave-safe bowl and cook in the microwave for about 1 minute.
3. Coat a small skillet with cooking spray and add the potatoes. Spritz lightly with cooking spray and cook over medium heat until brown.
4. While the potatoes are cooking, line a small baking tray with aluminum foil and lay the bacon strips flat. Cook in the pre-heated oven to desired crispiness, typically about 8-12 minutes.
5. When the potatoes are finished, move them to a serving plate and cook the egg in the same pan.
6. Arrange the plate with the potatoes, egg, and bacon. Add a small dollop of ketchup, if desired. (Make sure to add

in the calories for the ketchup, 5 calories per teaspoon.)

Preparation Notes:

Look for low-fat center cut bacon with about 23 calories per 5 g slice.

As an alternative to the grated potatoes, cook the potato in the microwave for a few minutes. Allow to cool, then cut into cubes. Cook in the skillet coated with spray oil until browned. Sprinkle with seasoned salt if desired.

Per Serving:

Calories	Fat	Carbohydrates	Protein	Sodium
175	4.5	19 g	12.5 g	250 mg

Mini Hash Brown Casseroles

Potatoes, if used sparingly, can be a great addition to fast days. The healthy, slow-release carbs provide energy throughout the morning.

Number of servings:	Serving size:	Calories per serving
3	2 mini casseroles	149

1 cup shredded potato, raw (about 1 medium potato)

½ cup minced onion (optional)

½ tsp. garlic powder

Salt and pepper

1 cup egg whites

¼ cup minced green pepper

1 oz. reduced-fat Swiss cheese

1 oz. ham, chopped

Cooking spray

Instructions:

1. *Preheat oven to 400 F.*
2. Spray a non-stick muffin pan with a generous amount of cooking spray.
3. Using a food processor or grater, shred the potato into narrow strips. Mix together with the onion, garlic powder, salt, and pepper.
4. Divide the potato mixture into 6 equal parts and scoop each part into one of the prepared muffin cups. Using the back of a spoon (or your fingers), press the potatoes along the sides and bottom of the pan to form a small cup or nest.
5. Bake the potatoes in the preheated oven for about 30 minutes or until golden brown.
6. While the potatoes are cooking, mix together the egg whites, green pepper, cheese, and ham.
7. When the potatoes are finished, remove the pan from the oven and fill each nest with egg white mixture.

8. Return the pan to the oven and bake until the eggs are fully cooked, about 20 minutes.

Preparation Notes:

If the potatoes stick to the muffin pan, try reusable silicone liners. Place a liner into each cup and spray lightly with cooking spray.

Experiment with other fillings! Instead of ham and green pepper, try:

- Chopped spinach and mushrooms (1/4 cup of each): reduces the calories per serving to 134.

- <u>Chicken-apple sausage</u> (1 patty), crumbled. No change to the calories per serving.

Per Serving:

Calories	Fat	Carbohydrates	Protein	Sodium
149	3 g	16 g	15 g	300 mg

Recipes: 200-300 Calories Per Serving

Some 5:2 dieters find that splitting their calories roughly evenly between breakfast and dinner is a workable strategy. But even if you prefer a smaller breakfast, these recipes are a great option for breakfast-for-dinner lovers.

Eggs Benedict (295 calories)

Overnight Oatmeal (295 calories)

Spicy Rice and Egg Bowl (266 calories)

Whole Wheat Banana Pancakes (258 calories)

Blueberry Oatmeal Pancakes (254 calories)

French Toast Waffles (256 calories)

Baked Apple Fritter (252 calories)

Omelet Wrap (225 calories)

Zucchini Breakfast Bread (235 calories)

Potato-Sausage Casserole (282 calories)

Eggs Benedict

A lower-calorie, lower-fat version of traditional Eggs Benedict, our recipes use a multi-grain muffin and a yogurt-based sauce.

Number of servings:	Serving size:	Calories per serving
1	1 portion	295

2 eggs

1 ounce Canadian bacon

1 <u>low-calorie, multi-grain English muffin</u>

2 Tbsp. plain Greek yogurt, fat-free

1 tsp. reduced fat mayonnaise

1 tsp. lemon juice

1 tsp. water

¼ tsp. dry mustard

Pinch of salt

Pinch of cayenne pepper

1 Tbsp. white vinegar

Parsley (for garnish)

Cooking spray

Instructions:

1. *In a small saucepan, whip together the yogurt, mayonnaise, lemon juice, water, mustard, salt, and pepper. Heat over low, stirring constantly, until well mixed and heated through. (Do not boil.) Remove pan from heat.*
2. Divide the Canadian bacon into two equal portions and cook in a small skillet (coat with cooking spray first). Heat for about 2 minutes per side then remove from heat and keep warm.
3. Split the English muffin and toast both halves.
4. Use a large skillet to poach the eggs (see Preparation Notes). *[Typically, eggs benedict is served with the yolks slightly runny; however consuming undercooked eggs may increase your risk of foodborne illness, especially if you have certain medical conditions.]*
5. To assemble, place the muffin halves onto a plate and top each with Canadian bacon. Add the poached eggs, and then slowly pour half of the sauce over each.

6. Garnish with parsley, if desired, and serve.

Preparation Notes:

How to poach an egg:

1. Fill a deep skillet with about two inches of water. Add 2 tsp. white vinegar and bring to a boil.
2. Reduce heat to low.
3. Crack the egg into a small bowl or cup without breaking the yolk, then gently pour into the water.
4. Use a spoon to move the egg whites close to the yolk.
5. Simmer for 4 minutes. Carefully spoon hot water over the yolk to help cook.
6. Lift the egg out of the pan with a slotted spoon.

For a change of taste, substitute asparagus, artichoke hearts, or spinach for the Canadian bacon. Revised calories are:

- 4 spears asparagus: 225 calories:

- ½ cup fresh spinach: 209 calories

- ½ cup artichoke hearts: 240 calories

Per Serving:

Calories	Fat	Carbohydrates	Protein	Sodium
295	12	27 g	22 g	950 mg

Overnight Oatmeal

Perfect for chilly mornings, make this the night before and wake up to a hot breakfast.

Number of servings:	Serving size:	Calories per serving
2	½ recipe	295

1 cup steel cut oats

3 Tbsp. brown sugar

½ tsp. salt

1 cup dried apricots, snipped into small pieces

3-1/2 cups water

1 cup fat-free buttermilk

1 tsp. vanilla

Cinnamon for dusting, if desired

Spray oil

Instructions:

1. *Spray a small slow cooker with oil.*
2. Mix the oats, sugar, and salt in a small bowl and pour into the slow cooker.
3. Layer the apricots on top of the oats.
4. Whip together the water, buttermilk, and vanilla, and pour into the slow cooker. Stir thoroughly.
5. Cover the slow cooker and set to low heat.
6. Cook for 7-8 hours without lifting the lid.
7. Dust with cinnamon and serve.

Preparation Notes:

Other dried fruits work well in this recipe, too. Substitute one of the following for the apricots:

¾ cup dried pears: 294 calories per serving

¾ cup dried apples: 279 calories per serving

½ cup dried banana: 291 calories per serving

½ cup dried cranberries: 268 calories per serving

Per Serving:

Calories	Fat	Carbohydrates	Protein	Sodium
295	4 g	56 g	10.5 g	750 mg

Spicy Rice and Egg Bowl

Another favorite from my California days, the whole grain provides the energy to help you last until dinner.

Number of servings:	Serving size:	Calories per serving
1	1 bowl	266

½ cup brown rice, cooked
¼ cup black beans (canned)
¼ cup corn (canned)
Salt

Black pepper

1 egg

2 Tbsp. salsa

1 small tomato, chopped

½ tsp. hot sauce

Spray oil

Instructions:
1. *Coat a medium skillet with oil and stir in the rice, beans, and corn. Sprinkle with salt and pepper and cook over low heat.*
2. While the rice mixture is heating, <u>poach the egg</u> in a separate skillet.
3. Spoon the rice into a bowl and top with the poached egg. Sprinkle with the chopped tomato and then pour on the salsa.
4. Drizzle with hot sauce and serve.

Preparation Notes:

If you're craving more of an Asian flair than Tex-Mex, heat the rice with ¼ cup frozen peas and 1-2 teaspoons of soy sauce (eliminate the beans, corn, tomato, salsa, and hot sauce.) Top the egg with a swirl of sriracha sauce. Prepared this way, the total calories are 228.

Per Serving:

Calories	Fat	Carbohydrates	Protein	Sodium
266	8 g	42.5 g	13.5 g	500 mg

Whole Wheat Banana Pancakes

A breakfast even non-dieters will love! With less than 260 calories per serving, you can drizzle lightly with maple syrup and still stay under budget.

Number of servings:	Serving size:	Calories per serving
4	3 3-inch pancakes	258

¾ cup whole wheat flour

½ cup all-purpose flour

2 Tbsp. sugar

1-½ tsp. baking powder

¼ tsp. salt

1 egg, lightly beaten

1 cup milk, fat-free

1 tsp. vanilla extract

1-½ medium bananas, diced (about 1-½ cups)

½ medium banana, sliced

Cooking spray

Instructions:

1. *Spray a non-stick griddle or skillet with cooking spray and heat over medium.*
2. Mix the flours together with the sugar, baking powder, and salt in a medium mixing bowl.
3. In a separate bowl, whisk together the egg, milk, and vanilla. Pour into the flour mixture and stir until the dry ingredients are just moistened. (Do not over stir or the pancakes will be dense and heavy.)
4. Fold the diced bananas into the batter.
5. Scoop a scant ¼ cup of batter per pancake onto the heated griddle. Cook about 2 minutes, or until bubbles form,

then flip. Continue cooking until golden brown.

6. To serve, place 3 pancakes per serving onto a plate and top with sliced bananas.

Preparation Notes:

For additional sweetness, drizzle each serving with ½ tablespoon of maple syrup (adds 26 calories per serving).

Per Serving:

Calories	Fat	Carbohydrates	Protein	Sodium
258	2 g	53 g	8 g	200 mg

Blueberry Oatmeal Pancakes

Oatmeal or pancakes? Why not have both! The slow-release energy from the whole grains is great for bridging the hours between breakfast and dinner.

Number of servings:	Serving size:	Calories per serving
4	3 3-inch	254

	pancakes	

¼ cup whole wheat flour
¼ cup all-purpose flour
¾ cup rolled oats (quick-cooking)
1 Tbsp. brown sugar
1 Tbsp. baking powder
¼ tsp. salt
1 egg
1 egg yolk
1 cup fat-free buttermilk
2 Tbsp. olive oil
1 tsp. vanilla extract
½ cup fresh or frozen blueberries
Handful of blueberries for topping
Cooking spray

Instructions:
1. *Spray a non-stick griddle or skillet with cooking spray and heat over medium.*
2. Mix the flours together with the oats, sugar, baking powder, and salt in a medium mixing bowl.

3. In a separate bowl, whisk together the egg, egg yolk, milk, olive oil, and vanilla. Pour into the flour mixture and stir until the dry ingredients are just moistened. (Do not over stir or the pancakes will be dense and heavy.)
4. Fold the blueberries into the batter.
5. Scoop a scant ¼ cup of batter per pancake onto the heated griddle. Cook about 2 minutes, or until bubbles form, then flip. Continue cooking until golden brown.
6. To serve, place 3 pancakes per serving onto a plate and top with a few berries.

Preparation Notes:

For even lower calories, replace the olive oil with 2 Tbsp. of applesauce (reduces the calories to 198 per serving). These have a tendency to stick to the griddle, however, so use a touch more cooking spray.

Per Serving:

Calories	Fat	Carbohydrates	Protein	Sodium

254	11	32 g	8 g	250 mg

French Toast Waffles

Another don't-make-me-choose option! Take traditional French toast and cook in a waffle maker for the best of both worlds.

Number of servings:	Serving size:	Calories per serving
2	2 waffles	256

2 eggs, lightly beaten

½ cup fat-free milk

1 Tbsp. sugar

1 tsp. vanilla extract

½ tsp. ground cinnamon

pinch of ground nutmeg

4 slices of bread, white or whole-wheat

Cooking spray

Instructions:

1. *Spray a waffle iron (preferably non-stick) with cooking spray and heat over medium.*
2. In a shallow bowl, whisk together the eggs, milk, sugar, vanilla, cinnamon, and nutmeg until well blended.
3. Dip the bread into the batter, coating both sides.
4. Place a battered slice into the waffle iron and close. Cook for about 6-8 minutes or until golden brown. (Since timing can vary, check after 5 minutes so they don't burn.)

Preparation Notes:

For ordinary white or whole wheat sandwich bread, a traditional square-shaped waffle maker works best.

Although ordinary white sugar works fine, "superfine" or caster sugar dissolves more easily for a more uniform batter.

The calorie counts are based on bread with 70 calories per slice.

For a low-calorie topping, sprinkle 1 tsp. powdered sugar onto 2 hot waffles, then squeeze a lemon wedge over it. Adds about 20 calories per serving.

Per Serving:

Calories	Fat	Carbohydrates	Protein	Sodium
256	5.5	40.5 g	11.5 g	350 mg

Baked Apple Fritter

When you want to indulge without going overboard, try this healthier take on a baked yeast doughnut.

Number of servings:	Serving size:	Calories per serving
4	1 fritter	252

¼ cup fat-free milk
¼ package active dry yeast
1-½ Tbsp. warm water
2 Tbsp. margarine, sliced
2 Tbsp. sugar
Pinch of salt

¼ cup whole wheat flour

½ cup all-purpose flour

½ tsp. cinnamon

1 egg

Spray oil

½ cup apple, peeled and chopped

½ cup powdered sugar

2 Tbsp. lemon juice

Instructions:

1. *Heat the milk over low-medium until scalding (about 100 F).*
2. While the milk is heating, dissolve the yeast into the warm water and allow to froth, about 5 minutes.
3. Stir together the margarine, sugar, and salt in a medium mixing bowl. Pour in the hot milk and allow the margarine to melt.
4. Stir in the whole wheat flour and mix well. Add the yeast mixture, cinnamon, and egg and stir until well blended.
5. Add the all-purpose flour and form into a dough.

6. Turn the dough onto a floured board and knead for several minutes. If the dough is too sticky sprinkle with additional flour. Form the dough into a ball.
7. Spray a mixing bowl with oil and add the dough. Spray the dough lightly, then cover the bowl with a clean cloth and place in a warm location for about 90 minutes.
8. When the dough has risen, punch it down and knead in the chopped apples. Divide into 4 equal portions and form each into a flattened sphere. Place on a baking sheet (spray with cooking spray first), cover lightly, and allow to rise for about 1 hour.
9. When the fritters have risen, bake in a pre-heated oven at 350°F for about 15 minutes or until golden brown.
10. While the dough is baking, mix the powdered sugar with the lemon juice and whisk until light and smooth to form the glaze.
11. Remove the fritters from the oven and brush with the glaze while still warm.

Per Serving:

Calories	Fat	Carbohydrates	Protein	Sodium
252	7.5	42.5 g	4.5 g	150 mg

Omelet Wrap

For a filling breakfast packed with flavor, this omelet wrap is a great option. Nice for lunch and dinner, too.

Number of servings:	Serving size:	Calories per serving
1	1 wrap	225

1 9-inch tortilla

2 egg whites

⅛ cup green pepper, chopped

1 Tbsp. green onion, chopped

1 Tbsp. fresh cilantro, chopped

½ tsp. hot sauce

2 Tbsp. prepared black bean dip (or 1/8 cup cooked black beans)

1 Tbsp. salsa

Cooking spray

Instructions:

1. *Whisk the egg whites and stir in the pepper, green onion, cilantro, and hot sauce.*
2. Coat a small skillet with cooking spray and cook the egg mixture.
3. While the eggs are cooking, place the tortilla between two paper towels and microwave for about 10 seconds.
4. Warm the bean dip (or beans) in the microwave, then spread onto the tortilla.
5. Scoop the cooked eggs onto the bean dip and spread evenly. Top with salsa and then roll the wrap.

Preparation Notes:

The calorie counts are based on tortillas with 150 calories each.

You can easily customize the filling to your liking. Pick and choose veggies from the table in Chapter 2 and adjust the calories accordingly.

Per Serving:

Calories	Fat	Carbohydrates	Protein	Sodium
225	3.5	34.5 g	14 g	900 mg

Zucchini Breakfast Bread

A low-calorie, whole wheat breakfast bread, great for when you need to eat and run.

Number of servings:	Serving size:	Calories per serving
10	1 slice (80 g)	235

1-½ cups whole wheat flour

½ cup sugar

¼ cup brown sugar

¼ tsp. baking soda

½ tsp. baking powder

¼ tsp. salt

1 tsp. cinnamon

½ tsp. nutmeg

2 eggs

2 medium zucchini, grated and drained (about 2-½ cups)

¼ cup canola oil

2 tsp. vanilla

½ cup walnuts, chopped

¼ cup candied ginger, chopped (optional)

Baking spray

Instructions:

1. *Preheat oven to 350 F.*
2. Spray a loaf pan (4" x 8") with baking spray.
3. Mix together the flour, sugar, baking soda, baking powder, salt, cinnamon, and nutmeg in a large mixing bowl.
4. In a separate bowl, whisk together the eggs, oil, and vanilla. Stir in the zucchini until well blended.
5. Pour the zucchini mixture into the flour mixture and stir well. Fold in the walnuts.
6. Pour the batter into the prepared loaf pan and bake for about 45 minutes

until a toothpick inserted into the center comes out clean.

Preparation Notes:

Drain the grated zucchini in a colander for at least 15 minutes before adding to the batter.

To lower the calories, replace the walnuts with dried (unsweetened) cranberries. This cuts out 30 calories per serving.

Per Serving:

Calories	Fat	Carbohydrates	Protein	Sodium
235	10.5 g	31.5 g	5 g	100 mg

Potato-Sausage Casserole

Perfect for weekend brunch, a single slice packs enough protein to last you most of the day.

Number of servings:	Serving size:	Calories per serving

| 8 | 1 slice (380 g) | 282 |

6 medium potatoes (about 2 pounds), peeled and diced

½ cup water

8 <u>low-calorie sausage patties</u>

6 eggs

8 egg whites

1 cup fat-free cottage cheese

½ cup parmesan cheese, grated

½ cup fat-free milk

2 Tbsp. dried parsley

½ tsp. salt

¼ tsp. black pepper

Cooking spray

Instructions:

1. *Preheat oven to 350 F.*
2. Spray a baking pan (9" x 13") with cooking spray.
3. Place the potatoes in a microwave-safe dish, add the water, and microwave

until soft, about 6 minutes. Drain thoroughly.

4. While the potatoes are cooking, spray a small skillet with cooking spray and pan fry the sausage over medium heat. Break up the patties into crumbles.
5. Add the potatoes to the prepared baking pan and spread evenly. Sprinkle with the sausage crumbles.
6. In a medium mixing bowl, stir together the eggs, egg whites, cottage cheese, parmesan, milk, parsley, salt, and pepper. Pour over the potatoes and sausage.
7. Bake the casserole in the preheated oven for about 45 minutes or until the top is golden brown and the center is set.
8. Cut into 8 slices and serve.

Preparation Notes:

For a lighter casserole, replace the sausage with 1 cup chopped broccoli (cooked) and ½ chopped red bell pepper. This reduces the calories per serving to 243.

Per Serving:

Calories	Fat	Carbohydrates	Protein	Sodium
282	8	30 g	26.5 g	650 mg

Conclusion

It is my sincere hope that you might have liked all the recipes which have been mentioned in the book and once again thank you for getting this book and experimenting with the recipes.

About The Author

Eduardo Pittman is born with the vision to promote *Intermittent fasting* among the masses. The author has written several research papers on the topic. He has served as an instructor promoting various cultural arts in University of San Francisco. He is currently living with his spouse in Texas.

CPSIA information can be obtained
at www.ICGtesting.com
Printed in the USA
BVHW041733161219
566813BV00021B/1838/P